Mediterranean Superfood Cookbook

100 Healthy and Delicious Mediterranean Recipes for a Low-Fat Diet

Olivia Armstrong

Copyright

Table of contents

- Spinach and mushroom quiche
- Mediterranean-style avocado toast

Chapter 3: Satisfying Soups and Salads

- Greek lentil soup
- Classic Greek salad with feta and olives
- Tuscan bean and vegetable soup
- Grilled chicken Caesar salad

Chapter 4: Wholesome Whole Grains

- Greek-style quinoa salad
- Mediterranean couscous with roasted vegetables
- Bulgur wheat and chickpea pilaf
- Lemon and herb brown rice

Chapter 5: Fantastic Fish and Seafood

- Grilled salmon with lemon and herbs
- Shrimp and vegetable skewers
- Baked cod with Mediterranean salsa

- Lentil and vegetable curry

Chapter 9: Mediterranean-Inspired Sides

- Tabbouleh salad
- Greek roasted potatoes
- Caprese skewers with balsamic glaze
- Grilled asparagus with lemon and garlic

Chapter 10: Sweet Mediterranean Treats

- Greek yogurt and honey parfait
- Orange and almond cake
- Baklava with pistachios and honey
- Fresh fruit salad with mint and yogurt dressing

Chapter 11: Beverages and Refreshments

- Mediterranean-style smoothies
- Mint and lemon infused water
- Greek frappé coffee
- Pomegranate and orange spritzer

Chapter 12: Weekly Meal Plans

- Sample meal plans for breakfast, lunch, and dinner
- Tips for meal prepping and planning ahead

Chapter 13: Tips for a Sustainable Mediterranean Lifestyle

- Incorporating physical activity into your routine
- Mindful eating practices
- Choosing locally sourced and seasonal ingredients
- Making the Mediterranean diet a long-term lifestyle

Chapter 1: Introduction to the Mediterranean Diet

Picture yourself strolling through a picturesque coastal village, the aroma of fresh herbs and olive oil wafting through the air, as you relish the vibrant colors and flavors of a Mediterranean feast. The Mediterranean diet, known for its delectable cuisine and numerous health benefits, has captured the hearts and taste buds of people around the world. In this chapter, we will embark on an exciting journey to unravel the secrets of the Mediterranean diet, its health benefits, guidelines for a low-fat Mediterranean diet, and the essential ingredients that make this culinary tradition so unique.

Understanding the Mediterranean Diet: More Than Just Food

The Mediterranean diet is not just another fad diet; it is a way of life. Originating from the countries surrounding the Mediterranean Sea, including Greece, Italy, Spain, and France, this dietary pattern has been celebrated for centuries for its contribution to longevity and overall well-being. At its core, the Mediterranean diet emphasizes whole, unprocessed foods, abundant fruits and vegetables, legumes, whole grains, lean proteins, and healthy fats. It is characterized by moderation, balance, and an appreciation for the pleasures of food.

Health Benefits of a Mediterranean Diet: A Fountain of Wellness

The health benefits associated with the Mediterranean diet are truly remarkable. Countless studies have shown that adhering to this dietary pattern can reduce the risk of chronic diseases and promote optimal health. One of the key benefits lies in its positive impact on heart health. The Mediterranean diet is rich in monounsaturated fats, found in olive oil, nuts, and avocados, which can lower LDL (bad) cholesterol levels and reduce the risk of heart disease.

Additionally, the Mediterranean diet is linked to a lower incidence of type 2 diabetes. The abundance of fiber-rich foods, such as whole grains, legumes, and vegetables, combined with the consumption of healthy fats, contributes to improved blood sugar control and insulin sensitivity.

Notably, the Mediterranean diet has been associated with a reduced risk of certain cancers, including breast, colorectal, and prostate cancers. The antioxidant-rich fruits and vegetables, along with the phytochemicals found in herbs and spices, exhibit powerful anti-inflammatory and cancer-fighting properties.

Guidelines for a Low-Fat Mediterranean Diet: Nourishing the Body, Savoring the Flavor

While the Mediterranean diet does include healthy fats, it is not an excuse for unlimited indulgence. For those seeking to follow a low-fat Mediterranean diet, there are some simple guidelines to keep in mind. Firstly, choose lean sources of protein, such as fish, poultry without skin, and legumes, while limiting red meat consumption. Secondly, opt for cooking methods that don't require excessive oil, such as grilling, baking, or steaming. Finally, moderation is key. While olive oil is an essential part of the Mediterranean diet, it's important to use it in moderation to maintain a low-fat approach.

Essential Ingredients in Mediterranean Cooking: Flavors that Dance on Your Palate

At the heart of Mediterranean cuisine are the incredible ingredients that create a symphony of flavors. Let's explore some of the staples you'll find in Mediterranean cooking:

Olive oil: The foundation of the Mediterranean diet, olive oil is rich in monounsaturated fats, antioxidants, and anti-inflammatory compounds. It is used for cooking, dressing salads, and adding a delightful richness to dishes.

Fresh fruits and vegetables: Bursting with vitamins, minerals, and fiber, fruits and vegetables take center stage in the Mediterranean diet. Tomatoes, peppers, eggplants, spinach, oranges, and figs are just a few of the abundant choices.

Whole grains: Nutrient-dense whole grains like barley, bulgur, farro, and whole wheat provide a hearty base for many

Mediterranean dishes. They offer a good source of fiber, vitamins, and minerals.

Legumes: From chickpeas and lentils to beans and peas, legumes are an excellent source of plant-based protein, fiber, and antioxidants. They are featured in soups, stews, salads, and spreads like hummus.

Fish and seafood: The Mediterranean Sea is teeming with an array of fish and seafood, including salmon, sardines, mackerel, shrimp, and octopus. These delicacies provide heart-healthy omega-3 fatty acids and lean protein.

Herbs and spices: Mediterranean cuisine relies on an assortment of herbs and spices to elevate flavors. Basil, oregano, rosemary, thyme, parsley, and cinnamon add depth and complexity to dishes without excessive salt or fat.

Nuts and seeds: Almonds, walnuts, pistachios, and sesame seeds are cherished ingredients in the Mediterranean diet. They offer healthy fats, protein, and a satisfying crunch to meals and snacks.

Conclusion: Embarking on a Flavorful Journey

As we conclude our introduction to the Mediterranean diet, we hope you're inspired to embark on a flavorful journey that will not only tantalize your taste buds but also promote your health and well-being. The Mediterranean diet is a testament to the fact that eating healthy doesn't have to be a sacrifice—it can be a celebration of life, food, and the joy of savoring each vibrant bite. So, gather your ingredients, fire up your stove, and get ready to explore the culinary wonders of the Mediterranean.

Chapter 2: Breakfast and Brunch Delights: Exploring the Mediterranean Morning Magic

Good morning, culinary adventurers! As the sun rises over the azure Mediterranean Sea, it brings with it a delightful spread of breakfast and brunch delights that will surely make your taste buds dance with joy. In this chapter, we dive into the world of Mediterranean morning magic, savoring the scrumptious creations that wake up our senses and energize our bodies for a day of adventure. From creamy yogurt parfaits to zesty omelets and indulgent quiches, get ready to experience breakfast like never before!

1. Greek Yogurt Parfaits with Fresh Fruits and Nuts: A Symphony of Creaminess and Crunch

Imagine a bowl filled with velvety Greek yogurt, crowned with a kaleidoscope of fresh fruits and adorned with a sprinkle of crunchy nuts. Welcome to the realm of Greek yogurt parfaits—a harmonious blend of textures and flavors that will leave you craving for more.

To assemble your parfait masterpiece, start with a generous dollop of thick and tangy Greek yogurt as the base. Then, layer on an assortment of colorful fruits like succulent strawberries, juicy blueberries, and vibrant kiwi slices. Each spoonful becomes a delightful journey as you encounter different fruity bursts.

But wait, there's more! Now, sprinkle some crunchy almond slivers, toasted walnuts, or honey-glazed pecans on top. These nuts not only add a delightful crunch but also provide a dose of healthy fats and essential nutrients.

The beauty of Greek yogurt parfaits is their versatility. Get creative and try different combinations of fruits and nuts to suit your taste preferences. For a tropical twist, add some sweet pineapple and shredded coconut. Or, for a more autumnal flair, layer in some diced apples, cinnamon, and a drizzle of maple syrup. The options are endless, and every creation will make your morning feel like a celebration.

2. Tomato and Feta Omelet: A Fluffy Pillow of Mediterranean Delight

As the sun climbs higher in the sky, let's turn up the heat on our stovetops and create a fluffy and flavorful Tomato and Feta Omelet. This Mediterranean classic is a simple yet satisfying way to start your day.

Begin by whisking together eggs, a splash of milk, and a pinch of salt and pepper. Pour the egg mixture into a preheated non-stick skillet and let it cook gently until the edges begin to set. Now, comes the star of the show—sweet and juicy tomatoes. Slice them into thin rounds and arrange them on one side of the omelet.

Next, crumble some creamy feta cheese over the tomatoes. The salty tang of the feta perfectly complements the sweetness of the tomatoes, creating a harmonious dance of flavors in your mouth.

Now, carefully fold the omelet in half, cocooning the tomatoes and feta inside. Let it cook for a few more minutes until the cheese starts to melt and the omelet turns a lovely golden hue.

Gently slide the omelet onto a plate, and there you have it—a fluffy pillow of Mediterranean delight ready to be devoured. Pair it with a side salad of mixed greens drizzled with a lemon-olive oil dressing, and you've got yourself a breakfast fit for a Greek god or goddess!

3. Spinach and Mushroom Quiche: A Hearty Brunch Marvel

Brunchtime calls for something a bit more indulgent, and that's where our Spinach and Mushroom Quiche steps into the spotlight. This delightful pastry creation is the perfect centerpiece for a leisurely brunch with friends and family.

Start by preparing the quiche crust. You can use a store-bought pie crust if you're short on time, or try your hand at making a flaky homemade crust from scratch. Once your crust is ready, it's time to dive into the savory filling.

In a sauté pan, cook a medley of earthy mushrooms and nutrient-rich spinach until they become tender and aromatic. Season them with a pinch of salt, pepper, and a sprinkle of nutmeg for that extra touch of warmth.

Now, whisk together eggs, milk, and a blend of your favorite cheeses—a combination of creamy feta, sharp cheddar, and nutty Gruyère works wonders. Pour the egg mixture over the spinach and mushrooms, allowing it to seep into every nook and cranny.

Bake the quiche in the oven until it turns a beautiful golden brown and the cheese melts into ooey-gooey goodness. The tantalizing aroma wafting through your kitchen will have everyone eagerly gathering around the table in anticipation.

Serve your Spinach and Mushroom Quiche with a side salad of mixed greens and cherry tomatoes drizzled with a balsamic vinaigrette. It's a hearty and wholesome brunch marvel that will impress your guests and leave them asking for the recipe.

4. Mediterranean-Style Avocado Toast: A Toast to Health and Happiness

Ah, avocado toast—the trendy sensation that has taken the breakfast world by storm. But let's put a Mediterranean twist on it to elevate this beloved classic to a whole new level of deliciousness.

Start with a thick slice of whole-grain bread, toasted to perfection. Spread a ripe avocado generously over the toast, using the back of a fork to create a creamy and luscious base.

Now comes the fun part—get creative with the toppings! We're talking about a Mediterranean fiesta here. Sprinkle some tangy crumbled feta, juicy cherry tomatoes, and a handful of briny Kalamata olives. Drizzle a touch of extra-virgin olive oil over the top, and if you're feeling adventurous, add a pinch of crushed red pepper flakes for a subtle kick.

One bite of this Mediterranean-style avocado toast, and you'll feel like you've been transported to a charming seaside café in the heart of Greece. The combination of creamy avocado, salty feta, and zesty tomatoes creates a harmonious symphony of flavors that will leave you feeling nourished and satisfied.

Conclusion: Savoring the Mediterranean Breakfast Bounty

As we bid farewell to this chapter filled with breakfast and brunch delights, we're reminded of the beauty and bounty that the Mediterranean diet brings to our mornings. From the creamy and crunchy Greek yogurt parfaits to the fluffy and flavorful Tomato and Feta Omelet, the hearty and wholesome Spinach and Mushroom Quiche, and the zesty and zingy Mediterranean-style Avocado Toast, the Mediterranean morning magic is a treasure trove of flavors and textures.

So, rise and shine with the Mediterranean breakfast delights on your plate, and let the spirit of the Mediterranean fill your day with health, happiness, and excitement for the next culinary adventure that awaits. Bon appétit!

Chapter 3: Satisfying Soups and Salads: A Symphony of Freshness and Flavor

Welcome to the world of hearty and satisfying soups and salads inspired by the sun-kissed Mediterranean. In this chapter, we'll dive into a delightful array of culinary creations that will tantalize your taste buds and leave you feeling nourished and satisfied. From the rich and comforting Greek lentil soup to the refreshing and vibrant Classic Greek salad, along with the soul-warming Tuscan bean and vegetable soup and the protein-packed Grilled Chicken Caesar salad, get ready for an adventure of flavors that will transport you straight to the shores of the Mediterranean!

1. Greek Lentil Soup: A Warm Hug in a Bowl

Picture this: a rustic pot of Greek lentil soup simmering on the stove, filling your home with the enticing aromas of onions, garlic, and fragrant herbs. As you ladle the steaming soup into bowls and take that first spoonful, you'll discover the heartiness and comfort that Greek lentil soup has to offer.

Start by sautéing onions, carrots, and celery until they become tender and slightly caramelized. This trio of vegetables forms the aromatic base of the soup, infusing it with depth and complexity.

Now, add in the star of the show—lentils. These tiny legumes are packed with protein, fiber, and essential nutrients, making them a wholesome and satisfying addition to any meal.

Cover the lentils and vegetables with a flavorful broth, and season generously with a medley of Mediterranean herbs like oregano, thyme, and bay leaves. A splash of lemon juice adds a burst of brightness to the soup, perfectly complementing the earthiness of the lentils.

As the soup simmers, the flavors meld together, creating a rich and velvety texture that warms both body and soul. To elevate this comforting dish, garnish it with a sprinkle of crumbled feta cheese and a drizzle of extra-virgin olive oil. The creamy feta adds a tangy note that balances the earthy lentils, while the olive oil imparts a silky richness that enhances every spoonful.

Serve your Greek lentil soup with a side of crusty bread, perfect for dipping into the savory broth. It's a bowl of warmth and nourishment that will make you feel like you've been wrapped in a cozy embrace.

2. Classic Greek Salad with Feta and Olives: A Symphony of Freshness

Let's transition from the warmth of the soup to the refreshing crispness of a Classic Greek salad. Bursting with vibrant colors and bold flavors, this salad is a true celebration of Mediterranean freshness.

Start with a bed of crisp romaine lettuce or mixed greens as the foundation of your salad. Then, layer on slices of succulent tomatoes and cucumbers, adding a juicy and refreshing element.

Now, let's introduce the stars of the show—Kalamata olives and creamy feta cheese. These iconic Mediterranean ingredients provide the salad with a delightful brininess and a luxurious richness that will transport your taste buds straight to the sun-drenched shores of Greece.

To enhance the flavors further, sprinkle some red onion slices and pepperoncini peppers over the salad. These add a hint of tanginess and a touch of spiciness, creating a symphony of tastes that dance on your palate.

To elevate the dressing, whisk together extra-virgin olive oil, red wine vinegar, dried oregano, and a pinch of salt and pepper. Drizzle this classic Greek dressing over the salad, and toss it gently to coat each ingredient with its tangy and herbaceous goodness.

The result? A Classic Greek salad that's as refreshing as a dip in the Mediterranean Sea. It's a perfect accompaniment to any meal, or you can make it the star of the show by adding some grilled chicken or shrimp for a more substantial and protein-packed option.

3. Tuscan Bean and Vegetable Soup: A Cozy Hug from Tuscany

As we continue our journey through the Mediterranean, let's make a stop in the heart of Tuscany, where the soul-warming Tuscan Bean and Vegetable Soup awaits.

This rustic and comforting soup showcases the bounty of seasonal vegetables, combined with creamy cannellini beans and a rich tomato broth. It's a celebration of simple, wholesome ingredients that come together to create a symphony of flavors.

To start, sauté a medley of chopped onions, carrots, and celery in a splash of olive oil until they become tender and fragrant. This trio of vegetables, known as the holy trinity of Italian cooking, forms the foundation of countless dishes in this region.

Next, add in canned or cooked cannellini beans, which are velvety and smooth, offering a delightful creaminess to the soup. Cannellini beans are not only rich in protein but also a good source of iron and fiber, making them a nutritious addition to your meal.

Now, it's time to introduce the star player—the tomatoes. Whether you choose to use canned tomatoes or fresh ones when they're in season, the tomatoes infuse the broth with a rich and robust flavor that ties all the ingredients together.

To enhance the taste even further, add a generous amount of Tuscan herbs, such as rosemary, thyme, and sage. These aromatic herbs contribute a delightful earthiness that makes you feel as though you're strolling through a Tuscan herb garden.

Let the soup simmer gently, allowing the flavors to meld and the vegetables to become tender. Just before serving, sprinkle some grated Parmesan cheese over the top and drizzle with a touch of extra-virgin olive oil. The cheese adds a salty kick, while the olive oil imparts a luxurious finish that will have you reaching for another bowl.

4. Grilled Chicken Caesar Salad: A Protein-Packed Mediterranean Delight

Last but not least, let's indulge in a Grilled Chicken Caesar Salad that combines the classic flavors of the Mediterranean with a protein-packed punch.

Start with tender and juicy grilled chicken breast, seasoned with a blend of Mediterranean herbs and a squeeze of lemon juice. Grilling the chicken not only enhances its flavor but also creates those coveted grill marks that add visual appeal to the dish.

Now, assemble the salad with a bed of fresh and crisp romaine lettuce. This vibrant leafy green provides a satisfying crunch and serves as the perfect canvas for the other ingredients.

Next, let's elevate the salad with the addition of croutons—crispy cubes of toasted bread that add a delightful texture contrast to the dish. You can make your own croutons by tossing cubes of day-old bread with olive oil and your favorite seasonings, then toasting them until golden and crunchy.

The pièce de résistance is the Caesar dressing. Whisk together creamy mayonnaise, tangy Dijon mustard, freshly squeezed lemon juice, minced garlic, and a generous grating of Parmesan cheese. The result is a velvety dressing with a perfect balance of creaminess and tanginess that coats the salad with a luscious embrace.

Toss the romaine lettuce and croutons in the Caesar dressing until each leaf is coated in its velvety goodness. Then, top the salad with slices of the grilled chicken breast, creating a protein-packed masterpiece that's both satisfying and delectable.

Conclusion: A Symphony of Mediterranean Flavors

As we conclude this chapter on Satisfying Soups and Salads, we're left with the lingering flavors

 of the Mediterranean—rich lentil soup, vibrant Greek salad, comforting Tuscan bean soup, and protein-packed Chicken Caesar salad. These culinary creations showcase the essence of Mediterranean cuisine, celebrating the freshness of ingredients, the harmony of flavors, and the nourishment of body and soul.

So, whether you're seeking a warm hug in a bowl or a refreshing burst of flavor on a plate, the Mediterranean has something to satisfy every craving. Join us on the next chapter of our culinary adventure as we explore more of the Mediterranean's treasures, from mouthwatering main courses to delectable desserts. Bon appétit!

Chapter 4: Wholesome Whole Grains: Elevating Flavor and Nutrition

Step into the world of Wholesome Whole Grains, where ancient grains take center stage, and vibrant flavors dance on your palate. In this chapter, we embark on a culinary journey that celebrates the nutritional power and delectable taste of whole grains in Mediterranean cuisine. From the protein-packed Greek-style Quinoa Salad to the aromatic Mediterranean Couscous with Roasted Vegetables, the hearty Bulgur Wheat and Chickpea Pilaf, and the zesty Lemon and Herb Brown Rice, get ready to be amazed by the magic of whole grains in every delightful bite!

1. Greek-style Quinoa Salad: A Protein-Packed Powerhouse

First on our whole grain adventure is the Greek-style Quinoa Salad—a nutritional powerhouse that delights both vegans and omnivores alike. Quinoa, pronounced "keen-wah," has taken the culinary world by storm due to its high protein content and nutty flavor profile.

To create this masterpiece, start by cooking quinoa in vegetable broth, which imparts a savory depth to the grains. Once the quinoa is tender and fluffy, let it cool slightly before assembling the salad.

In goes the medley of fresh Mediterranean vegetables—diced cucumbers, juicy cherry tomatoes, tangy red onions, and crisp bell peppers—all adding vibrant colors and a refreshing crunch.

But that's not all! To elevate the flavors even further, toss in some briny Kalamata olives and crumbled feta cheese. These Mediterranean treasures bring a delightful salty and tangy dimension to the salad, making each bite an explosion of taste.

Finally, dress the salad with a simple yet zesty vinaigrette made with extra-virgin olive oil, freshly squeezed lemon juice, minced garlic, and a pinch of dried oregano. This dressing complements the nutty quinoa and fresh vegetables, tying the whole salad together in a harmonious symphony of flavors.

2. Mediterranean Couscous with Roasted Vegetables: A Satisfying Melody of Textures

Next up is the Mediterranean Couscous with Roasted Vegetables—a dish that showcases the versatility and adaptability of couscous, a traditional North African grain made from durum wheat semolina.

To prepare this comforting dish, start by roasting an array of vegetables—sweet bell peppers, earthy eggplant, zucchini, and juicy cherry tomatoes—tossed in a medley of Mediterranean herbs, such as thyme, rosemary, and basil. As the vegetables roast in the oven, their flavors intensify, creating a medley of aromas that will leave your kitchen smelling like a culinary paradise.

Meanwhile, prepare the couscous by simply soaking it in hot vegetable broth until it fluffs up into tender, bite-sized grains. The couscous acts as a canvas, ready to absorb the flavors of the roasted vegetables and the herb-infused broth.

When the vegetables are beautifully caramelized and tender, toss them with the couscous, creating a delightful marriage of textures and flavors. Each mouthful is a satisfying melody of chewy couscous, velvety vegetables, and aromatic herbs.

For a finishing touch, drizzle some extra-virgin olive oil over the couscous, and sprinkle a handful of toasted pine nuts or almond slivers on top. These crunchy additions provide the perfect contrast to the tender couscous and add a touch of richness to the dish.

3. Bulgur Wheat and Chickpea Pilaf: A Hearty and Wholesome Harmony

Now, let's venture into the realm of hearty pilafs with the Bulgur Wheat and Chickpea Pilaf. Bulgur wheat, a staple in Middle Eastern and Mediterranean cuisines, is a whole grain that has been parboiled and cracked, making it a quick-cooking and nutritious option.

To start this pilaf, sauté onions and garlic in a bit of olive oil until they become golden and aromatic. Then, add the bulgur wheat to the pan, toasting it slightly to enhance its nutty flavor.

Next, add cooked chickpeas to the mix. Chickpeas, also known as garbanzo beans, are not only a great source of plant-based protein but also add a creamy and hearty texture to the pilaf.

Now comes the time to infuse the pilaf with a blend of Mediterranean spices. A pinch of cumin, a dash of cinnamon, and a sprinkle of ground coriander create a tantalizing aroma that transports you to the bustling markets of the Mediterranean.

Cover the mixture with vegetable broth, and let it simmer until the bulgur wheat absorbs all the flavors and becomes tender. This process infuses the pilaf with a medley of spices and creates a harmonious blend of ingredients.

To serve, fluff up the pilaf with a fork and garnish it with a handful of chopped fresh parsley or cilantro. These herbs not only add a burst of color but also provide a refreshing contrast to the earthy flavors of the bulgur and chickpeas.

4. Lemon and Herb Brown Rice: A Citrusy Sensation

Last but certainly not least, let's explore the world of Lemon and Herb Brown Rice—a zesty and aromatic creation that puts a Mediterranean twist on a classic grain.

Begin by cooking brown rice in a mixture of vegetable broth and water, which infuses the grains with savory goodness. Brown rice, with its outer bran intact, offers a nutty flavor and a chewier texture compared to its white rice counterpart. Plus, it's packed with fiber and essential nutrients, making it a nutritious choice for any meal.

As the rice cooks, prepare a flavorful dressing by whisking together extra-virgin olive oil, freshly squeezed lemon juice, minced garlic, and a generous amount of chopped fresh herbs, such as parsley, dill, and mint. This lemon and herb dressing adds a bright and citrusy note to the rice, elevating its flavor profile to new heights.

Once the rice is tender and fluffy, gently fold in the lemon and herb dressing, ensuring that every grain is coated in its zesty goodness. The result is a bowl of brown rice that's anything but ordinary—it's a citrusy sensation that will keep you coming back for more.

Conclusion: A Symphony of Whole Grain Delights

As we conclude this chapter on Wholesome Whole Grains, we are left with a symphony of flavors that celebrate the nutritional power and delectable taste of these ancient grains. From the protein-packed Greek-style Quinoa Salad to the aromatic Mediterranean Couscous with Roasted Vegetables, the hearty Bulgur Wheat and Chickpea Pilaf, and the zesty Lemon and Herb Brown Rice, each dish takes us on a journey through the Mediterranean, where freshness, harmony, and nourishment come together in every delightful bite.

So, venture into the world of whole grains, and let their magic transform your culinary adventures into something truly extraordinary. Whether you're seeking a comforting bowl of pilaf or a refreshing grain salad, whole grains offer a plethora of options to elevate your meals to new heights of flavor and nutrition. Let the Mediterranean's bounty of grains inspire you, and continue exploring the culinary treasures that await in the chapters ahead. Bon appétit!

Chapter 5: Fantastic Fish and Seafood: A Journey into Oceanic Delights

Ahoy, food adventurers! Prepare to set sail on a culinary voyage that explores the bountiful treasures of the sea. In this chapter, we dive into the world of Fantastic Fish and Seafood, where succulent flavors and oceanic delights await. From the sizzling Grilled Salmon with Lemon and Herbs to the delightful Shrimp and Vegetable Skewers, the delectable Baked Cod with Mediterranean Salsa, and the hearty Seafood Paella, get ready to be swept away by the mouthwatering magic of the ocean.

1. Grilled Salmon with Lemon and Herbs: A Symphony of Sizzle

Our first stop takes us to the sizzling shores of Grilled Salmon with Lemon and Herbs. Salmon, with its rich pink flesh and buttery texture, is a true ocean gem that captivates seafood lovers worldwide.

To embark on this flavor-packed journey, start by creating a zesty marinade. Whisk together freshly squeezed lemon juice, fragrant minced garlic, a drizzle of extra-virgin olive oil, and a medley of aromatic herbs, such as dill, thyme, and rosemary. This marinade infuses the salmon with a delightful tang and herbal goodness, creating a melody of flavors that dance on your taste buds.

Allow the salmon to bask in the marinade for at least 30 minutes, letting the magic happen as the flavors meld together. Then, it's time to hit the grill!

As the salmon sizzles over the flames, the aroma of lemon and herbs fills the air, tantalizing your senses. Each side of the salmon develops a delicious char, sealing in its moistness and enhancing its succulent taste.

Once the salmon is cooked to perfection, garnish it with fresh sprigs of dill, a sprinkle of lemon zest, and a pinch of sea salt. This finishing touch elevates the dish to new heights of visual and culinary delight.

Serve your Grilled Salmon with Lemon and Herbs with a side of roasted vegetables or a vibrant Greek salad. It's a dish fit for a coastal feast that celebrates the wonders of the ocean.

2. Shrimp and Vegetable Skewers: A Colorful Kabob Fiesta

Next, we sail towards the delightful world of Shrimp and Vegetable Skewers—a colorful kabob fiesta that celebrates the marriage of succulent shrimp and vibrant vegetables.

To begin this culinary adventure, marinate the plump shrimp in a citrusy blend of lemon juice, garlic, olive oil, and a hint of smoky paprika. Let the shrimp luxuriate in this tangy bath, absorbing all the flavors that will make them burst with taste.

Now, it's time to thread the shrimp onto skewers along with an array of colorful vegetables. Imagine juicy cherry tomatoes, crisp bell peppers, zucchini slices, and red onions—all beautifully arranged on the skewers.

The kabobs are ready to hit the grill, where the shrimp turn pink and tender, and the vegetables become slightly charred, releasing their natural sweetness.

As the skewers sizzle on the grill, the scent of grilled shrimp and vegetables drifts through the air, creating an enticing aroma that beckons you to the table.

Once cooked, slide the Shrimp and Vegetable Skewers onto a platter and garnish with a sprinkle of chopped fresh parsley or cilantro. These herbs provide a burst of freshness and add a final touch of color to the dish.

Serve your kabob fiesta with a side of couscous, rice, or pita bread. It's a wholesome and festive meal that invites everyone to savor the delights of the sea and land.

3. Baked Cod with Mediterranean Salsa: A Wholesome Symphony of Flavors

Our culinary voyage now leads us to the Baked Cod with Mediterranean Salsa—a wholesome symphony of flavors that celebrates the bounty of the Mediterranean.

Start by seasoning the cod fillets with a blend of Mediterranean herbs, such as oregano, thyme, and basil. This herbal infusion elevates the mild flavor of the cod, transforming it into a Mediterranean masterpiece.

Place the seasoned cod fillets in a baking dish and top them with a generous spoonful of Mediterranean salsa. This vibrant and colorful salsa is a medley of diced tomatoes, briny Kalamata olives, tangy capers, chopped fresh basil, and a drizzle of extra-virgin olive oil.

As the cod bakes in the oven, it becomes tender and flaky, while the Mediterranean salsa intensifies in flavor, creating a taste symphony that will transport you straight to the shores of Italy or Greece.

Garnish your Baked Cod with Mediterranean Salsa with lemon wedges and a sprinkle of chopped parsley. The lemon adds a burst of citrusy brightness, while the parsley adds a final touch of freshness.

Serve this delightful dish with a side of quinoa or couscous, soaking up the savory juices of the salsa. It's a wholesome and nourishing meal that brings the vibrant flavors of the Mediterranean to your table.

4. Seafood Paella: A Hearty Feast for the Senses

Last but not least, our culinary journey culminates in the grand finale of Seafood Paella—a hearty feast for the senses that captures the essence of Spanish cuisine.

In a traditional paella pan, sauté a symphony of flavors—onions, garlic, bell peppers, and tomatoes. This aromatic base sets the stage for the indulgent flavors that will follow.

Now, add in the star of the show—saffron-infused rice. Saffron, known as "red gold," imparts a distinct golden hue and a delicate floral aroma to the rice, making it a luxurious ingredient in this dish.

Pour in a rich seafood broth, allowing the rice to soak up all the savory goodness. The seafood broth forms the backbone of the paella, infusing every grain of rice with flavor and richness.

Now, it's time to add a medley of seafood treasures—plump shrimp, tender squid, succulent mussels, and flavorful clams. Nestle the seafood into the rice, creating a stunning tapestry of colors and textures.

As the paella simmers, the aroma of saffron and seafood wafts through the air, creating an atmosphere of excitement and anticipation.

Once the rice has absorbed all the flavors and the seafood is cooked to perfection, it's time to savor the masterpiece. Serve your

Seafood Paella with wedges of lemon and a sprinkle of chopped fresh parsley.

Gather around the table, and let the paella be the center of attention as friends and family dive into the luscious blend of rice and seafood. It's a festive and indulgent meal that celebrates the splendor of the sea and the joy of sharing a memorable feast.

Conclusion: A Symphony of Oceanic Delights

As we conclude this chapter on Fantastic Fish and Seafood, we find ourselves enchanted by the tantalizing tastes of the ocean. From the sizzling Grilled Salmon with Lemon and Herbs to the delightful Shrimp and Vegetable Skewers, the delectable Baked Cod with Mediterranean Salsa, and the hearty Sea food Paella, each dish takes us on a culinary voyage that celebrates the ocean's bounty and the artistry of Mediterranean cuisine.

So, set sail on your own culinary adventure and discover the magic of fish and seafood in creating flavorful and wholesome meals. Whether you prefer the sizzle of the grill, the zesty burst of salsa, or the indulgence of a paella feast, the oceanic delights of this chapter offer something special for every palate. Let the flavors of the sea captivate you, and continue exploring the culinary treasures that await in the chapters ahead. Bon appétit!

Chapter 6: Poultry and Lean Meat Marvels: A Sizzling Symphony of Flavors

Prepare to indulge in a sizzling symphony of flavors as we journey into the world of Poultry and Lean Meat Marvels. In this chapter, we explore the delectable creations that celebrate the succulence of poultry and the wholesome goodness of lean meats. From the zesty Lemon and Garlic Chicken Skewers to the aromatic Moroccan Spiced Turkey Meatballs, the succulent Grilled Lamb Chops with Mint Yogurt Sauce, and the mouthwatering Italian-style Turkey Breast with Roasted Vegetables, get ready to be dazzled by the magic of these savory delights!

1. Lemon and Garlic Chicken Skewers: A Citrusy Fiesta

Our culinary adventure begins with a citrusy fiesta of Lemon and Garlic Chicken Skewers.

Imagine succulent chunks of chicken, marinated in a tangy blend of fresh lemon juice, fragrant garlic, and a hint of smoky paprika.

To create this mouthwatering masterpiece, start by cutting boneless chicken breast into bite-sized pieces. Then, whisk together the marinade—zesty lemon juice, minced garlic, a drizzle of extra-virgin olive oil, and a pinch of paprika for that delightful hint of smokiness.

Let the chicken bask in the marinade for at least 30 minutes, allowing the flavors to infuse and transform the chicken into a tender and flavorful delight.

Once marinated, thread the chicken pieces onto skewers, ready to be sizzled to perfection on the grill. As the skewers cook, the lemon and garlic aroma fills the air, creating an enticing ambiance that makes everyone eager to dig in.

When the chicken is cooked to juicy perfection and lightly charred, it's time to feast! Serve your Lemon and Garlic Chicken Skewers with a side of colorful salad or fluffy couscous. It's a zesty and satisfying dish that will brighten up any mealtime.

2. Moroccan Spiced Turkey Meatballs: An Aromatic Adventure

Next, we venture into the aromatic world of Moroccan Spiced Turkey Meatballs—an exotic delight that tantalizes the senses with a medley of spices.

Start by combining lean ground turkey with a fragrant blend of Moroccan spices—cumin, coriander, cinnamon, and a touch of cayenne pepper for a subtle kick. These warm and earthy spices create an irresistible aroma that whisks you away to the bustling spice markets of Morocco.

Form the seasoned turkey mixture into bite-sized meatballs, ready to be baked to perfection in the oven. As the meatballs cook, the kitchen fills with a tantalizing scent that stirs the appetite and promises a savory adventure.

Meanwhile, prepare a delightful yogurt sauce infused with fresh mint, garlic, and a squeeze of lemon juice. This cooling and tangy sauce complements the spiced meatballs, creating a harmonious balance of flavors.

Once the meatballs are golden brown and aromatic, serve them alongside the mint yogurt sauce, inviting your guests to drizzle it generously over the meatballs. The combination of warm spices and cooling yogurt creates a symphony of tastes that transports your taste buds to a Moroccan feast.

3. Grilled Lamb Chops with Mint Yogurt Sauce: A Heavenly Treat

Now, our culinary journey takes us to a heavenly treat—Grilled Lamb Chops with Mint Yogurt Sauce. Lamb chops, with their tender texture and robust flavor, are a gourmet indulgence that's sure to impress.

To begin this succulent adventure, marinate the lamb chops in a blend of Mediterranean herbs, such as rosemary, thyme, and oregano, along with garlic and a drizzle of olive oil. This aromatic marinade infuses the lamb with a symphony of flavors that intensify as the chops grill to perfection.

As the lamb chops sizzle on the grill, their tantalizing aroma fills the air, making your mouth water with anticipation. Each side develops a beautiful char, sealing in the juiciness and enhancing the succulence of the meat.

While the lamb chops grill, prepare a refreshing mint yogurt sauce. Combine tangy Greek yogurt with fresh mint leaves, minced garlic, and a hint of lemon zest. This creamy and cooling sauce is the perfect accompaniment to the rich flavors of the lamb.

Once the lamb chops are cooked to your desired doneness, serve them on a platter, garnished with a sprinkle of fresh mint leaves. The lamb chops, accompanied by the mint yogurt sauce, create a heavenly pairing that's fit for a feast.

4. Italian-style Turkey Breast with Roasted Vegetables: A Wholesome Delight

Our final stop on this culinary adventure leads us to the wholesome delight of Italian-style Turkey Breast with Roasted Vegetables. Lean turkey breast, marinated with Italian herbs and roasted to perfection, creates a meal that's both comforting and nutritious.

Start by marinating the turkey breast in a blend of Italian herbs, such as basil, oregano, and thyme, along with garlic and a drizzle of olive oil. This herb-infused marinade enhances the flavor of the turkey and transports you to the sun-drenched landscapes of Italy.

Allow the turkey breast to soak in the marinade for at least an hour, letting the flavors infuse and make the meat tender and aromatic.

Meanwhile, prepare a colorful medley of vegetables—sweet bell peppers, zucchini, cherry tomatoes, and red onions—tossed in a light coat of olive oil and seasoned with a touch of salt and pepper.

Roast the turkey breast and vegetables together in the oven, creating a hearty and wholesome meal that fills your home with the aroma of an Italian feast.

Once the turkey breast is cooked to perfection and the vegetables are tender and slightly caramelized, serve them on a platter, ready to be savored.

Conclusion: A Sizzling Symphony of Poultry and Lean Meat Marvels

As we conclude this chapter on Poultry and Lean Meat Marvels, we find ourselves enthralled by the sizzling symphony of flavors that celebrate the succulence of poultry and the wholesomeness of lean meats.

From the citrusy fiesta of Lemon and Garlic Chicken Skewers to the aromatic adventure of Moroccan Spiced Turkey Meatballs, the heavenly treat of Grilled Lamb Chops with Mint Yogurt Sauce, and the wholesome delight of Italian-style Turkey Breast with

Roasted Vegetables, each dish brings its own unique magic to the table.

So, savor the succulence and indulge in the savory goodness of poultry and lean meats. Whether you're grilling, baking, or roasting, the marvels of this chapter offer something delightful for every palate. Let the flavors whisk you away to distant lands and continue exploring the culinary wonders that await in the chapters ahead. Bon appétit!

Chapter 7: Bountiful Vegetable Dishes: A Garden of Delightful Flavors

Welcome to the enchanting world of Bountiful Vegetable Dishes, where the freshest produce takes center stage and vibrant flavors dance on your taste buds. In this chapter, we embark on a culinary journey that celebrates the wholesome goodness and delectable taste of vegetables. From the delightful Ratatouille with Fresh Herbs to the savory Stuffed Bell Peppers with Quinoa and Feta, the indulgent Eggplant Parmesan, and the comforting Roasted Mediterranean Vegetables, get ready to be amazed by the magic of these vegetable delights!

1. Ratatouille with Fresh Herbs: A Symphony of Garden Goodness

Our culinary adventure begins with the symphony of flavors that is Ratatouille with Fresh Herbs. This classic French dish showcases a medley of seasonal vegetables, cooked to perfection and infused with the aroma of fresh herbs.

To create this delightful masterpiece, start by slicing eggplants, zucchini, bell peppers, and tomatoes into uniform rounds. These colorful and wholesome vegetables are the stars of the show, each contributing its unique flavor and texture to the dish.

In a large pot or skillet, sauté onions and garlic until they become fragrant and slightly caramelized. This forms the aromatic base of the ratatouille, creating a foundation of flavors that will elevate the dish to new heights.

Now, add the sliced vegetables to the pot, arranging them in a beautiful and overlapping pattern. The key to a stunning ratatouille is the presentation, where the colors and shapes of the vegetables create a visually appealing garden on your plate.

Next, sprinkle a generous amount of fresh herbs, such as basil, thyme, and rosemary, over the vegetables. These fragrant herbs infuse the ratatouille with a burst of garden goodness, making each bite a delightful celebration of flavors.

Cover the pot and let the ratatouille simmer gently until the vegetables become tender and absorb the herb-infused flavors. The result is a luscious and comforting dish that pays tribute to the bounty of the garden.

Serve your Ratatouille with Fresh Herbs with a side of crusty bread or over a bed of fluffy couscous. It's a dish that captures the essence of seasonal vegetables and celebrates the simple joys of home-cooked goodness.

2. Stuffed Bell Peppers with Quinoa and Feta: A Wholesome Fiesta

Next, we venture into a wholesome fiesta of flavors with Stuffed Bell Peppers with Quinoa and Feta. These colorful and vibrant bell peppers are filled with a delightful mixture of quinoa and creamy feta cheese, creating a satisfying and nutritious meal.

To begin this culinary adventure, cook quinoa in vegetable broth until it becomes light and fluffy. Quinoa, a protein-packed grain, offers a nutty taste and a wholesome texture that complements the sweetness of the bell peppers.

In a mixing bowl, combine the cooked quinoa with crumbled feta cheese, diced tomatoes, chopped fresh parsley, and a drizzle of olive oil. This mixture forms the heart of the stuffed bell peppers, infusing them with a symphony of flavors.

Now, slice the tops off the bell peppers and remove the seeds and membranes to create a hollow cavity. Stuff each bell pepper with the quinoa and feta mixture, generously filling them to create a bountiful feast.

As the stuffed bell peppers bake in the oven, their aroma fills the air, beckoning everyone to the table. The quinoa and feta mixture becomes slightly golden and develops a delightful crust, adding a satisfying crunch to each bite.

Once the stuffed bell peppers are tender and slightly charred, serve them on a platter, garnished with a sprinkle of fresh parsley or cilantro. The combination of quinoa, feta, and bell peppers creates a wholesome fiesta that celebrates the vibrant flavors of the garden.

3. Eggplant Parmesan: An Indulgent Italian Delight

Now, our culinary journey leads us to the indulgent delight of Eggplant Parmesan—a classic Italian dish that celebrates the richness of eggplant and the comfort of melted cheese.

To create this luscious masterpiece, start by slicing eggplant into thin rounds and seasoning them with a pinch of salt. This step draws out any excess moisture from the eggplant, ensuring a crisp and delicious result.

Dip the seasoned eggplant slices into a mixture of beaten eggs and milk, then coat them with a blend of breadcrumbs and grated Parmesan cheese. This breading adds a delightful crunch and savory richness to the eggplant.

Fry the breaded eggplant slices until they become golden and crispy, infusing your kitchen with the enticing aroma of comfort food.

Now comes the fun part—layering the eggplant with marinara sauce and mozzarella cheese. In a baking dish, spread a generous amount of marinara sauce, then arrange a layer of fried eggplant slices over the sauce. Top the eggplant with a layer of mozzarella cheese, creating a cheesy and savory embrace.

Repeat the layers until all the eggplant is used, finishing with a final layer of sauce and mozzarella on top. The result is a bubbling and indulgent delight that's as comforting as a warm hug.

Bake the Eggplant Parmesan in the oven until the cheese melts and becomes beautifully golden. The eggplant absorbs the rich flavors of the sauce and cheese, creating a heavenly marriage of textures and tastes.

Once the Eggplant Parmesan is cooked to perfection, serve it on a platter, garnished with a sprinkle of fresh basil leaves. The crispy eggplant, gooey cheese, and zesty marinara sauce come together in a mouthwatering symphony that's perfect for sharing with loved ones.

4. Roasted Mediterranean Vegetables: A Comforting Classic

Our final stop on this vegetable adventure leads us to the comforting classic of Roasted Mediterranean Vegetables—a dish that celebrates the simplicity and flavors of the Mediterranean.

To create this comforting masterpiece, toss a colorful medley of vegetables—zucchini, red onions, cherry tomatoes, and bell peppers—with a generous drizzle of olive oil. The olive oil not only enhances the flavors of the vegetables but also helps them caramelize and become slightly charred during roasting.

Sprinkle the vegetables with a medley of Mediterranean herbs, such as thyme, oregano, and basil, along with a pinch of salt and pepper. These aromatic herbs infuse the vegetables with a delightful aroma and create a harmonious blend of flavors.

Roast the vegetables in the oven until they become tender and slightly caramelized, releasing their natural sweetness and creating an irresistible aroma that fills your home with comfort.

Once roasted to perfection, serve the Mediterranean vegetables on a platter, ready to be savored. This versatile dish pairs beautifully with grilled meats, fish, or even on its own as a wholesome and satisfying vegetarian meal.

Conclusion: A Garden of Delightful Flavors

As we

conclude this chapter on Bountiful Vegetable Dishes, we find ourselves enchanted by the garden of delightful flavors that celebrate the wholesome goodness and delectable taste of vegetables.

From the symphony of garden goodness in Ratatouille with Fresh Herbs to the wholesome fiesta of Stuffed Bell Peppers with Quinoa and Feta, the indulgent delight of Eggplant Parmesan, and the comforting classic of Roasted Mediterranean Vegetables, each dish brings its own unique magic to the table.

So, savor the freshness and indulge in the savory goodness of vegetables. Whether you're simmering, stuffing, roasting, or baking, the marvels of this chapter offer something delightful for every palate. Let the flavors whisk you away to a garden of culinary delights and continue exploring the wonders that await in the chapters ahead. Enjoy!

Chapter 8: Delectable Legume Creations: A World of Flavorful Delights

Get ready to embark on a culinary adventure that celebrates the humble yet mighty legumes. In this chapter, we explore the delectable Legume Creations that take us on a journey across the Mediterranean and beyond. From the creamy Classic Greek Hummus to the hearty Tuscan White Bean Soup, the exotic Chickpea and Vegetable Tagine, and the flavorful Lentil and Vegetable Curry, get ready to be amazed by the magic of these legume delights!

1. Classic Greek Hummus: Creamy and Tangy

Our culinary journey begins with a creamy and tangy delight—the Classic Greek Hummus. This Mediterranean gem, made from humble chickpeas, celebrates simplicity and flavor.

To create this mouthwatering masterpiece, start by blending cooked chickpeas with tahini (a paste made from sesame seeds), fresh lemon juice, garlic, and a drizzle of olive oil. The result is a smooth and velvety dip that's rich in flavor and oh-so-creamy.

Imagine dipping a warm pita bread or crisp vegetable sticks into the luscious hummus, savoring the blend of nutty tahini, zesty lemon, and the subtle kick of garlic. It's a party for your taste buds!

Garnish the hummus with a drizzle of extra-virgin olive oil, a sprinkle of paprika, and a few whole chickpeas. This final touch not only adds a burst of color but also enhances the flavors, making every bite a delight.

2. Tuscan White Bean Soup: Hearty and Comforting

Next, we venture to the heart of Tuscany to savor the Hearty Tuscan White Bean Soup. This rustic and comforting dish showcases the wholesome goodness of white beans in a medley of aromatic flavors.

To begin this culinary journey, cook white beans until they become tender and creamy. Imagine the beans absorbing the flavors of aromatic herbs, garlic, and a savory vegetable broth.

Now, add a medley of vegetables—carrots, celery, and tomatoes—to the pot, creating a colorful tapestry that brings the soup to life.

The aroma of simmering soup fills the air, promising a comforting and nourishing feast. With each spoonful, you taste the richness of the beans, the sweetness of the vegetables, and the harmony of the herbs.

Serve your Tuscan White Bean Soup with a sprinkle of grated Parmesan cheese and a few fresh basil leaves. The cheese adds a savory depth, while the basil provides a refreshing note that elevates the flavors.

3. Chickpea and Vegetable Tagine: Exotic and Flavorful

Now, we set sail to North Africa to savor the Exotic Chickpea and Vegetable Tagine—a tantalizing stew that combines the earthiness of chickpeas with a melody of aromatic spices.

To create this flavor-packed delight, sauté onions, garlic, and a blend of Moroccan spices—cumin, coriander, and cinnamon—in a fragrant tagine or a large pot.

Imagine the scent of spices filling the kitchen, transporting you to the bustling markets of Marrakech.

Add chickpeas, sweet potatoes, carrots, and tomatoes to the pot, creating a vibrant and colorful mix of ingredients.

As the tagine simmers, the vegetables become tender, and the chickpeas soak up the exotic flavors of the spices.

The result is a savory and wholesome dish that's as beautiful as it is delicious.

Serve your Chickpea and Vegetable Tagine with a side of fluffy couscous, allowing it to soak up the flavorful broth. The combination of chickpeas, vegetables, and spices creates a symphony of tastes that transport you to the heart of Morocco.

4. Lentil and Vegetable Curry: Spicy and Satisfying

Last but not least, our culinary journey takes us to the aromatic Lentil and Vegetable

Curry—a dish that celebrates the boldness of lentils and the warmth of Indian spices.

To begin this flavorful adventure, cook lentils until they become tender and velvety. Imagine the lentils absorbing the flavors of ginger, garlic, and a blend of Indian spices—turmeric, cumin, and garam masala.

Now, add a medley of vegetables—bell peppers, spinach, and cauliflower—to the pot, creating a colorful and nutrient-rich curry.

As the curry simmers, the lentils meld with the spices, and the vegetables become vibrant and aromatic.

The result is a spicy and satisfying dish that warms your soul and nourishes your body.

Serve your Lentil and Vegetable Curry with a side of fluffy basmati rice or warm naan bread. The combination of lentils, vegetables, and spices creates a symphony of tastes that takes you on a culinary journey to the heart of India.

Conclusion: A World of Flavorful Delights

As we conclude this chapter on Delectable Legume Creations, we find ourselves enchanted by the magic of these humble yet mighty ingredients.

From the creamy Classic Greek Hummus to the hearty Tuscan White Bean Soup, the exotic Chickpea and Vegetable Tagine, and the flavorful Lentil and Vegetable Curry, each dish takes us on a culinary adventure that celebrates the diverse and vibrant world of legumes.

So, savor the creaminess of hummus, the heartiness of white beans, the exotic spices of tagine, and the warmth of lentils. Whether you're dipping, stewing, or simmering, the legume creations in this chapter offer a world of flavorful delights that cater to every palate.

Let the magic of legumes inspire you, and continue exploring the culinary wonders that await in the chapters ahead.

Chapter 9: Mediterranean-Inspired Sides: A Symphony of Flavors

Prepare to tantalize your taste buds with a symphony of flavors as we delve into the world of Mediterranean-Inspired Sides. In this chapter, we explore a delightful array of dishes that perfectly complement any meal. From the refreshing Tabbouleh Salad to the crispy Greek Roasted Potatoes, the elegant Caprese Skewers with Balsamic Glaze, and the vibrant Grilled Asparagus with Lemon and Garlic, get ready to elevate your dining experience with these Mediterranean-inspired delights!

1. Tabbouleh Salad: A Refreshing Herb-infused Delight

Our culinary adventure begins with the refreshing Tabbouleh Salad—a vibrant dish that celebrates the essence of Mediterranean flavors and fresh herbs.

Imagine a medley of finely chopped fresh parsley, juicy tomatoes, crisp cucumbers, and tangy lemon juice, all tossed together with bulgur wheat. This salad is a celebration of textures, colors, and the invigorating taste of herbs.

The aromatic herbs, such as mint and parsley, lend a refreshing and vibrant note, while the lemon juice adds a tangy kick that brightens the entire dish.

As you take a bite, the combination of the crisp vegetables, the nuttiness of bulgur wheat, and the herb-infused dressing create a delightful dance on your palate. It's a perfect side dish that complements grilled meats or seafood, adding a burst of freshness to every bite.

2. Greek Roasted Potatoes: Crispy and Flavorful

Next, we travel to Greece to savor the crispy and flavorful delight of Greek Roasted Potatoes—a side dish that brings a taste of the Mediterranean to your table.

Picture golden-brown potatoes, perfectly crispy on the outside and tender on the inside. These roasted potatoes are infused with the flavors of olive oil, lemon juice, garlic, and aromatic herbs, such as oregano and thyme.

To create this culinary masterpiece, toss the potato wedges with the herb-infused marinade and let them soak up the flavors for a while. As they roast in the oven, the enticing aroma fills your kitchen, building anticipation for the satisfying crunch that awaits.

Once roasted to perfection, the potatoes are a symphony of textures and flavors. Each bite reveals a crispy exterior that gives way to a fluffy and flavorful center.

Serve your Greek Roasted Potatoes as a side dish to grilled meats, fish, or even as part of a mezze platter. They are a delightful accompaniment that transports you to the sun-drenched shores of the Mediterranean.

3. Caprese Skewers with Balsamic Glaze: A Bite-sized Delight

Now, we turn our attention to an elegant and bite-sized delight—Caprese Skewers with Balsamic Glaze. This classic Italian dish showcases the simplicity of fresh ingredients in a stunning presentation.

Imagine plump cherry tomatoes, creamy mozzarella cheese, and fresh basil leaves, all threaded onto skewers. This colorful and flavorful combination creates a visually appealing appetizer or side dish that captures the essence of Mediterranean cuisine.

To elevate the flavor profile, drizzle the skewers with a balsamic glaze—a sweet and tangy reduction of balsamic vinegar. The glaze adds a touch of sophistication and complements the freshness of the ingredients.

As you take a bite, the burst of juicy tomatoes, the creamy mozzarella, the aromatic basil, and the tangy balsamic glaze create a harmonious and irresistible combination. Each skewer is a delightful explosion of flavors in your mouth.

Serve your Caprese Skewers with Balsamic Glaze as an appetizer or side dish at your next gathering, and watch as your guests indulge in this elegant and refreshing Mediterranean-inspired treat.

4. Grilled Asparagus with Lemon and Garlic: Vibrant and Zesty

Our final stop on this Mediterranean-inspired culinary journey takes us to Grilled Asparagus with Lemon and Garlic—a vibrant and zesty side dish that celebrates the freshness of asparagus.

Imagine tender asparagus spears, perfectly grilled to bring out their natural sweetness and smoky flavors. These charred beauties are then tossed with a tangy dressing of fresh lemon juice, fragrant garlic, and a drizzle of extra-virgin olive oil.

As you take a bite, the bright and crisp asparagus, with its slightly smoky notes, blends harmoniously with the zesty citrus and the savory garlic. The combination creates a delightful balance of flavors that adds vibrancy to any meal.

Serve your Grilled Asparagus with Lemon and Garlic alongside grilled meats, fish, or as part of a Mediterranean-inspired salad. It's a versatile and refreshing side dish that adds a touch of elegance to any table.

Conclusion: A Symphony of Mediterranean-Inspired Sides

As we conclude this chapter on Mediterranean-Inspired Sides, we find ourselves captivated by the symphony of flavors that elevate any meal to new heights.

From the refreshing Tabbouleh Salad to the crispy Greek Roasted Potatoes, the elegant Caprese Skewers with Balsamic Glaze, and the vibrant Grilled Asparagus with Lemon and Garlic, each dish showcases the freshness, vibrancy, and simplicity that make Mediterranean cuisine so captivating.

So, add a touch of the Mediterranean to your table with these delightful sides.

Whether you're enjoying a casual meal or hosting a gathering, the flavors and textures of these dishes will transport you to the sun-kissed shores of the Mediterranean.

Chapter 10: Sweet Mediterranean Treats: A Journey to Sweet Paradise

Welcome to Chapter 10: Sweet Mediterranean Treats! Brace yourself for a delightful journey to sweet paradise as we explore a delectable array of desserts inspired by the Mediterranean. From the luscious Greek Yogurt and Honey Parfait to the zesty Orange and Almond Cake, the indulgent Baklava with Pistachios and Honey, and the refreshing Fresh Fruit Salad with Mint and Yogurt Dressing, each treat is a masterpiece that will satisfy your sweet cravings and transport you to the enchanting world of Mediterranean flavors.

1. Greek Yogurt and Honey Parfait: Creamy Bliss with a Touch of Sweetness

Let's kick off this sweet journey with the luscious Greek Yogurt and Honey Parfait—a creamy and delightful treat that celebrates the simplicity and richness of Greek yogurt.

Imagine layers of velvety Greek yogurt, drizzled with a golden stream of honey. Each spoonful is a harmony of smoothness and sweetness that will leave you craving for more.

To add a delightful twist, top your parfait with a sprinkle of chopped nuts, such as toasted almonds or walnuts. These crunchy additions offer a textural contrast that elevates the parfait to new heights.

Indulge in the Greek Yogurt and Honey Parfait as a guilt-free dessert or a satisfying breakfast treat. It's a celebration of Mediterranean goodness that's as wholesome as it is delicious.

2. Orange and Almond Cake: Zesty Citrus Bliss

Next on our sweet adventure, we encounter the Orange and Almond Cake—a zesty delight that combines the bright flavors of oranges with the nutty goodness of almonds.

Imagine a moist and fragrant cake, infused with the citrusy aroma of freshly squeezed orange juice and zest. The almond meal adds a delightful richness and texture that makes each bite irresistible.

The cake is a celebration of harmony between sweet and tangy flavors. Each slice is a burst of zesty citrus bliss that pairs beautifully with a cup of tea or coffee.

As you savor the Orange and Almond Cake, let its delightful aroma and bright flavors transport you to the sun-kissed orchards of the Mediterranean, where orange groves thrive and almond trees sway in the breeze.

3. Baklava with Pistachios and Honey: Irresistible Indulgence

Now, prepare to be enchanted by the Baklava with Pistachios and Honey—a legendary Mediterranean treat that is the epitome of indulgence.

Imagine layers of delicate phyllo pastry, generously brushed with melted butter and sprinkled with a luscious mixture of ground pistachios and aromatic spices.

Each layer is a symphony of flavors, creating a crispy and nutty sensation that melts in your mouth.

Once baked to golden perfection, the Baklava is drizzled with a sweet and fragrant honey syrup, infusing every morsel with a touch of sweetness.

As you take a bite, the combination of flaky pastry, crunchy pistachios, and luscious honey creates an irresistible indulgence that will have you reaching for more.

The Baklava with Pistachios and Honey is not just a dessert; it's a work of art that pays tribute to the rich culinary heritage of the Mediterranean. Savor it with friends and family, and let the flavors transport you to the bustling markets and charming cafes of the Mediterranean.

4. Fresh Fruit Salad with Mint and Yogurt Dressing: A Refreshing Symphony

Our final stop on this sweet journey brings us to the refreshing Fresh Fruit Salad with Mint and Yogurt Dressing—a delightful symphony of juicy fruits, aromatic mint, and creamy yogurt.

Imagine a bowl filled with a colorful assortment of fresh fruits, such as sweet strawberries, succulent peaches, tangy kiwis, and ripe blueberries. Each fruit offers its unique sweetness and vibrant hue, creating a visual feast.

To elevate the flavors, drizzle the fruit salad with a dressing made from creamy Greek yogurt, honey, and a sprinkle of fresh mint leaves.

As you take a spoonful, the medley of fruits, the coolness of yogurt, and the refreshing burst of mint create a harmonious combination that refreshes your senses.

The Fresh Fruit Salad with Mint and Yogurt Dressing is not only a dessert but also a healthy and wholesome option to satisfy your sweet tooth. It's a celebration of the bountiful produce of the Mediterranean, where fresh fruits thrive under the sun.

Conclusion: A Journey to Sweet Paradise

As we conclude Chapter 10: Sweet Mediterranean Treats, we hope you are enchanted by the flavors and indulgence of these delightful desserts.

From the creamy Greek Yogurt and Honey Parfait to the zesty Orange and Almond Cake, the indulgent Baklava with Pistachios and Honey, and the refreshing Fresh Fruit Salad with Mint and Yogurt Dressing, each sweet treat offers a unique and exciting experience for your taste buds.

So, embrace the sweetness of the Mediterranean and let these delightful desserts transport you to a world of pure indulgence and bliss.

Continue your culinary journey and discover the treasures that await in the upcoming chapters. Bon appétit and sweet travels!

Chapter 11: Beverages and Refreshments: Quench Your Thirst with Mediterranean Magic

Welcome to Chapter 11: Beverages and Refreshments! Get ready to quench your thirst with a taste of Mediterranean magic. In this exciting chapter, we explore a delightful array of beverages and refreshments that capture the essence of the Mediterranean lifestyle. From the invigorating Mediterranean-Style Smoothies to the revitalizing Mint and Lemon Infused Water, the bold Greek Frappé Coffee, and the vibrant Pomegranate and Orange Spritzer, each drink is a masterpiece that will elevate your drinking experience and transport you to the sun-kissed shores of the Mediterranean.

1. Mediterranean-Style Smoothies: A Burst
of Freshness

Let's start our beverage adventure with the
invigorating Mediterranean-Style
Smoothies—a burst of freshness that
celebrates the bountiful produce of the
Mediterranean.

Imagine a blender filled with a colorful
assortment of fresh fruits, such as ripe
strawberries, luscious peaches, and tangy
oranges. Add a handful of creamy Greek
yogurt, a splash of honey, and a drizzle of
olive oil for a touch of Mediterranean flair.

As the blender whirls into action, the
vibrant colors and enticing aroma fill the air,
promising a delightful treat for your taste
buds.

Each sip of the Mediterranean-Style
Smoothies is a celebration of freshness and
nourishment. The combination of juicy

fruits, creamy yogurt, and the smooth richness of olive oil creates a delightful symphony of flavors that will keep you coming back for more.

Indulge in these smoothies for a wholesome breakfast, a midday pick-me-up, or a post-workout treat. They are not only delicious but also a great way to kickstart your day with a burst of energy and vitality.

2. Mint and Lemon Infused Water: Revitalize Your Senses

Next, we encounter the revitalizing Mint and Lemon Infused Water—a simple yet refreshing beverage that will revitalize your senses and quench your thirst.

Imagine a jug filled with cold water, adorned with sprigs of fresh mint and slices of zesty lemon. The water absorbs the invigorating flavors of mint and lemon, creating a beverage that's as delightful to look at as it is to taste.

As you take a sip, the coolness of the water, the refreshing burst of mint, and the zing of lemon create a revitalizing sensation that hydrates and invigorates your body.

The Mint and Lemon Infused Water is a perfect companion for hot summer days or after a challenging workout. It's a celebration of simplicity and the natural goodness of Mediterranean herbs and fruits.

Keep a jug of this infused water on your table and let its invigorating flavors uplift your spirits and keep you refreshed throughout the day.

3. Greek Frappé Coffee: Bold and Frothy

Now, prepare to be captivated by the bold and frothy Greek Frappé Coffee—a classic

Mediterranean treat that's a favorite among coffee enthusiasts.

Imagine a tall glass filled with ice, topped with a frothy layer of coffee and creamy milk. The Greek Frappé Coffee is an artful combination of instant coffee, sugar, water, and ice, whipped to perfection into a delightful foam.

As you take your first sip, the bold flavor of the coffee, the creaminess of the milk, and the frothy texture create a sensational experience that's both satisfying and invigorating.

The Greek Frappé Coffee is not just a drink—it's a cultural phenomenon that brings people together in cafes and on sunny terraces. It's a celebration of leisure and the joy of savoring every moment.

Sip on this delightful coffee during a laid-back afternoon or as a delightful pick-me-up in the morning. It's a drink that captures the spirit of the Mediterranean lifestyle—relaxed, vibrant, and full of flavor.

4. Pomegranate and Orange Spritzer: Vibrant and Effervescent

Our final stop on this beverage journey brings us to the vibrant and effervescent Pomegranate and Orange Spritzer—a delightful concoction that combines the bold flavors of pomegranate and orange with a splash of sparkling water.

Imagine a tall glass filled with crushed ice, topped with the vibrant hues of pomegranate juice and freshly squeezed orange juice. Add a splash of sparkling water, and watch as the bubbles dance and infuse the drink with effervescence.

As you take a sip, the tangy sweetness of the pomegranate, the zesty brightness of the orange, and the refreshing fizz of the sparkling water create a sensational burst of flavors on your palate.

The Pomegranate and Orange Spritzer is not only a refreshing beverage but also a celebration of Mediterranean fruits and the joy of summer.

Savor this effervescent spritzer during a leisurely brunch or as a delightful companion to a Mediterranean-inspired meal. It's a drink that adds a touch of vibrancy to any occasion and elevates your drinking experience to new heights.

Conclusion: Quench Your Thirst with Mediterranean Magic

As we conclude Chapter 11: Beverages and Refreshments, we hope you are enchanted by the magical

flavors and refreshing delights of the Mediterranean.

From the invigorating Mediterranean-Style Smoothies to the revitalizing Mint and Lemon Infused Water, the bold Greek Frappé Coffee, and the vibrant Pomegranate and Orange Spritzer, each drink is a masterpiece that captures the essence of the Mediterranean lifestyle—vibrant, refreshing, and full of zest.

So, embrace the magic of Mediterranean beverages and let these delightful treats transport you to the sun-drenched shores and charming cafes of the Mediterranean.

Continue your culinary journey and discover the treasures that await in the upcoming chapters. Cheers and here's to your next adventure in the world of Mediterranean flavors!

Chapter 12: Weekly Meal Plans: Fuel Your Week with Delicious Delicacies

Welcome to Chapter 12: Weekly Meal Plans! Get ready to embark on a journey of culinary delights as we explore sample meal plans for breakfast, lunch, and dinner. Whether you're a seasoned chef or a kitchen novice, these meal plans will ignite your taste buds and inspire your creativity in the kitchen. From energizing breakfasts to satisfying lunches and delightful dinners, we've got you covered for the entire week. And, to make your life easier, we'll share some invaluable tips for meal prepping and planning ahead, so you can enjoy delicious meals without the stress!

Sample Meal Plan 1: A Mediterranean Morning

Breakfast:

- Mediterranean-Style Smoothie: Kickstart your day with a burst of freshness. Blend ripe strawberries, creamy Greek yogurt, and a drizzle of honey for a delightful treat that's as nutritious as it is delicious.

Lunch:
- Greek Lentil Salad: Savor the flavors of the Mediterranean with this hearty salad. Combine cooked lentils, juicy cherry tomatoes, crisp cucumbers, and tangy feta cheese. Drizzle with olive oil and a squeeze of lemon juice for an irresistible lunch.

Dinner:
- Lemon and Garlic Chicken Skewers: Transport yourself to the Mediterranean with these flavorful chicken skewers. Marinate chunks of chicken in a zesty lemon and garlic dressing, then grill to perfection. Serve with a side of Greek Roasted Potatoes for a satisfying dinner.

Sample Meal Plan 2: Coastal Delights

Breakfast:
- Orange and Almond Cake: Indulge in the zesty goodness of oranges and the nutty richness of almonds with this delightful cake. Enjoy a slice with your morning coffee or tea for a sweet start to your day.

Lunch:
- Caprese Skewers with Balsamic Glaze: Elevate your lunchtime with these elegant and bite-sized treats. Thread cherry tomatoes, fresh mozzarella, and basil leaves onto skewers, then drizzle with balsamic glaze for a burst of flavor.

Dinner:
- Grilled Salmon with Lemon and Herbs: Treat yourself to a taste of the coast with succulent grilled salmon. Season with fresh herbs, lemon zest, and a pinch of sea salt for a refreshing and healthy dinner.

Sample Meal Plan 3: A Taste of the Mediterranean

Breakfast:
- Tabbouleh Salad: Start your day with a refreshing twist on the classic salad. Prepare a batch of Tabbouleh Salad the night before, and enjoy it as a light and nourishing breakfast.

Lunch:
- Greek Frappé Coffee: Sip on the bold and frothy Greek Frappé Coffee for a delightful midday pick-me-up. It's the perfect companion to keep you energized and refreshed.

Dinner:
- Pomegranate and Orange Spritzer: End your day with a vibrant and effervescent drink. The Pomegranate and Orange Spritzer is a delightful way to relax and unwind after a long day.

Tips for Meal Prepping and Planning Ahead

1. Create a Weekly Meal Plan: Take some time at the beginning of each week to plan your meals. Consider your schedule, preferences, and any special occasions that may affect your meals. Write down a list of breakfast, lunch, and dinner options for each day of the week.

2. Shop Smart: Once you have your meal plan ready, create a shopping list with all the ingredients you'll need. Stick to your list when you go grocery shopping to avoid impulse purchases and ensure you have everything you need for the week.

3. Prep in Advance: Take advantage of downtime during the week to do some meal prepping. Chop vegetables, marinate meats, or prepare sauces ahead of time. This will save you time and make cooking during the week much easier.

4. Batch Cooking: Consider cooking larger quantities of certain dishes that can be used for multiple meals. For example, prepare a big batch of lentil salad that can be enjoyed for lunch over several days.

5. Mix and Match: Be flexible with your meal plans. If you have leftover ingredients from one meal, try incorporating them into another dish to minimize food waste and add variety to your meals.

6. Freeze for Later: If you have leftovers that you won't be able to finish within a few days, freeze them for later. This way, you'll have ready-made meals on hand for those busy days when cooking from scratch is not an option.

7. Stay Inspired: Keep a collection of your favorite recipes and meal ideas for future reference. Experiment with new flavors and cuisines to keep your meals exciting and enjoyable.

Conclusion: A Week of Culinary Delights

As we conclude Chapter 12: Weekly Meal Plans, we hope you're excited to fuel your week with delicious delicacies and creative culinary adventures. With these sample meal plans and tips for meal prepping and planning ahead, you'll breeze through your week with a satisfied palate and a happy heart.

So, embrace the joy of meal planning and discover the wonders of the Mediterranean-inspired cuisine. Whether you're indulging in Mediterranean-Style Smoothies, savoring Lemon and Garlic Chicken Skewers, or enjoying a refreshing Pomegranate and Orange Spritzer, each meal is a celebration of flavors and a journey to culinary bliss.

Continue exploring the delights that await in the upcoming chapters and remember to

always have fun in the kitchen. Bon appétit
and happy meal planning!

Chapter 13: Tips for a Sustainable Mediterranean Lifestyle: Embrace a Vibrant and Balanced Way of Living

Welcome to Chapter 13: Tips for a Sustainable Mediterranean Lifestyle! Get ready to dive into the essence of the Mediterranean way of living—a lifestyle that promotes overall well-being, sustainability, and a strong connection with nature. In this exciting chapter, we'll explore practical tips to incorporate physical activity into your routine, practice mindful eating, choose locally sourced and seasonal ingredients, and make the Mediterranean diet a long-term lifestyle. So, let's embark on this journey of embracing a vibrant and balanced way of living that nourishes both your body and soul!

1. Incorporating Physical Activity into Your Routine: Move with Joy

In the Mediterranean, physical activity is not seen as a chore but as a joyful part of daily life. From strolling along picturesque coastal paths to dancing to traditional music, movement is a celebration of vitality and connection.

Tip 1: Embrace Nature's Playground
Take advantage of your natural surroundings. Whether you're walking in the park, hiking through the woods, or swimming in the sea, immerse yourself in the beauty of nature while staying active.

Tip 2: Find Joy in Movement
Choose activities that bring you joy. From dancing to gardening, find ways to move that make you feel happy and alive. Physical activity should never be a burden but a delightful expression of your energy.

Tip 3: Make it Social
Engage in physical activities with friends and family. Whether it's playing a game of soccer or going for a group hike, shared experiences strengthen bonds while keeping you active.

2. Mindful Eating Practices: Savor Every Bite

The Mediterranean way of eating is not just about what you eat but how you eat. Mindful eating is a key aspect of this lifestyle, helping you fully appreciate and savor your meals.

Tip 1: Slow Down and Savor
Take your time to enjoy each meal. Put away distractions, such as phones and TVs, and focus on the flavors and textures of your food. Eating slowly allows your body to recognize when it's full, preventing overeating.

Tip 2: Engage All Senses
Engage all your senses when eating. Observe the colors, smell the aromas, feel the textures, and savor the tastes. This multisensory experience enhances your connection with the food.

Tip 3: Respect Your Hunger and Fullness
Listen to your body's hunger and fullness cues. Eat when you're hungry and stop when you're satisfied. Avoid eating out of boredom or emotions and practice self-awareness around your eating habits.

3. Choosing Locally Sourced and Seasonal Ingredients: Nourish the Planet and Yourself

The Mediterranean diet places great importance on fresh and seasonal ingredients. By choosing locally sourced foods, you support local farmers, reduce your carbon footprint, and enjoy produce at its peak.

Tip 1: Visit Farmers' Markets
Explore your local farmers' markets and discover an abundance of fresh and seasonal produce. Engage with the farmers and learn about the origins of your food.

Tip 2: Plant a Garden
Consider starting a small garden, even if it's just a few herbs on your windowsill. Growing your own food fosters a deeper connection with nature and provides a sense of accomplishment.

Tip 3: Rediscover Forgotten Foods
Explore ancient grains, heirloom vegetables, and traditional ingredients. Rediscover forgotten foods that are not only nutritious but also part of your cultural heritage.

4. Making the Mediterranean Diet a Long-Term Lifestyle: A Journey of Flavorful Wellness

The Mediterranean diet is not a short-term fad; it's a way of life. Embrace the journey of flavorful wellness and commit to nourishing your body and soul with the goodness of this lifestyle.

Tip 1: Start Small and Build Gradually
Implementing lifestyle changes can be overwhelming. Start by incorporating one or two Mediterranean-inspired meals into your weekly routine, and gradually expand from there.

Tip 2: Discover New Recipes
Explore the vast array of Mediterranean recipes available. Experiment with different ingredients and cooking methods to keep your meals exciting and varied.

Tip 3: Cultivate a Positive Mindset
Approach the Mediterranean lifestyle with a positive and open mindset. Embrace the journey with enthusiasm and curiosity,

knowing that every step is a step towards greater well-being.

Conclusion: Embrace a Vibrant and Balanced Way of Living

As we conclude Chapter 13: Tips for a Sustainable Mediterranean Lifestyle, we hope you're inspired to embrace this vibrant and balanced way of living.

Incorporating physical activity into your routine, practicing mindful eating, choosing locally sourced and seasonal ingredients, and making the Mediterranean diet a long-term lifestyle are all steps towards nurturing your body, soul, and the planet.

Embrace the joy of movement, savor the flavors of your meals, and connect with the rhythms of nature. Let the Mediterranean lifestyle nourish your well-being and infuse every aspect of your life with vitality and delight.

Continue exploring the wonders of Mediterranean-inspired living and remember that each small step is a part of the beautiful journey towards a more sustainable and fulfilling life. Bon voyage on your exciting path to a vibrant and balanced lifestyle!